Fit at 60: The Ultimate Guide to Workout for seniors over 60

Louisa Smith

Table of content

Introduction

As we age, our bodies undergo many changes, and it becomes increasingly important to prioritize our health and fitness. Staying active and maintaining a healthy lifestyle is crucial for seniors over 60 to prevent or manage chronic conditions, maintain mobility, and promote overall wellbeing.

However, many seniors are unsure of where to start when it comes to exercise. There are so many different workout programs, machines, and classes available, and it can be overwhelming to decide what is right for your body and fitness level.

That's where "Fit at 60: The Ultimate Guide to Workout for Seniors over 60" comes in. This guide is designed to provide seniors with all the information they need to develop a safe, effective workout routine tailored to their individual needs.

First and foremost, this guide emphasizes the importance of consulting with a healthcare professional before starting any new exercise program. As we age, we are more susceptible to injury and health complications, so it's crucial to make sure that our bodies are ready for exercise and that we don't have any underlying health conditions that could be exacerbated by physical activity.

Once you have the green light from your doctor, the guide dives into the different types of exercise that are best for seniors over 60. It's important to choose activities that are low-impact and easy on the joints, such as walking, swimming, cycling, and yoga. These exercises are not only safe but also provide a range of health benefits, including improved cardiovascular health, increased strength and flexibility, and reduced risk of falls.

The guide also includes information on strength training, which is especially important for seniors to maintain muscle mass and prevent age-related muscle loss. However, strength training should be approached with caution, as seniors are more susceptible to injury and may have existing joint or muscle pain. The guide provides tips for selecting the right exercises and equipment, as well as advice on how to gradually increase weight and intensity to prevent injury.

In addition to exercise, the guide emphasizes the importance of nutrition and hydration for seniors over 60. As we age, our bodies require different nutrients and may be less efficient at processing food and absorbing nutrients. It's important to make sure that we are getting enough protein, fiber, and vitamins, and staying hydrated to support our overall health and fitness.

The guide also provides tips for staying motivated and making exercise a habit. It can be challenging to stick to a new workout routine, especially if you have not been active in a while. However, there are many strategies that can help, such as setting achievable goals, finding a workout partner, and keeping track of progress.

Finally, "Fit at 60" addresses some common concerns and misconceptions around exercise for seniors. For example, many seniors worry that exercise is not safe or effective for them, or that they will not be able to keep up with younger, fitter individuals in group classes or at the gym. However, these concerns are often unfounded, and the guide provides reassurance and practical advice for seniors looking to get active.

In summary, "Fit at 60: The Ultimate Guide to Workout for Seniors over 60" is an essential resource for anyone looking to improve their health and fitness in their golden years. Whether you are a seasoned athlete or just starting out with exercise, this guide provides practical advice, expert insights, and motivational tips to help you achieve your fitness goals and maintain a healthy, active lifestyle.

Chapter 1

Benefits of Exercising for Seniors Over 60

Regular exercise is important for people of all ages, but it becomes even more crucial as we get older. For seniors over 60, exercise can offer numerous health benefits, both physical and mental. Here are some of the key benefits of exercising for seniors over 60:

Improved cardiovascular health: Regular exercise can help seniors maintain healthy blood pressure and cholesterol levels, which can reduce their risk of heart disease and stroke.

Increased strength and mobility: Strength training and other types of exercise can help seniors build and maintain muscle mass, which can improve their balance, coordination, and mobility.

Better bone health: Weight-bearing exercises can help seniors maintain strong bones and reduce their risk of osteoporosis and fractures.

Reduced risk of chronic diseases: Regular exercise can help prevent or manage chronic conditions such as diabetes, arthritis, and certain types of cancer.

Improved mental health: Exercise can help seniors reduce stress, improve their mood, and boost their cognitive function, including memory and attention.

Increased social interaction: Exercise can provide seniors with an opportunity to socialize and connect with others, which can improve their overall sense of well-being.

Overall, regular exercise is essential for seniors over 60 to maintain their physical and mental health and enjoy a high quality of life. It's important for seniors to choose exercises that are safe and appropriate for their level of fitness and any underlying health conditions they may have.

When choosing exercises, seniors should take into account their current fitness level, any health conditions they may have, and any physical limitations they may experience. It's important to start slowly and gradually increase the duration and intensity of their workouts. Seniors should also consult with their doctor before starting any new exercise program.

Importance of Stretching for Seniors Over 60

Stretching is an important component of any exercise routine, especially for seniors over 60. Stretching can improve flexibility, reduce the risk of injury, and help seniors maintain their mobility and independence. Here are some of the key benefits of stretching for seniors over 60:

Improved flexibility: Stretching exercises can help seniors improve their flexibility and range of motion, which can reduce the risk of joint pain and stiffness.

Reduced risk of injury: Stretching before and after exercise can help seniors warm up and cool down their muscles, reducing the risk of muscle strains and other injuries.

Increased blood flow: Stretching can help improve circulation and blood flow to the muscles, which can reduce muscle soreness and fatigue.

Improved posture: Stretching exercises can help seniors improve their posture and reduce the risk of back pain and other musculoskeletal issues.

Reduced stress: Stretching can help seniors reduce stress and tension in their muscles, which can improve their overall sense of well-being.

Seniors can incorporate stretching into their exercise routine by doing simple stretches such as shoulder rolls, neck stretches, and hamstring stretches. They should hold each stretch for 15-30 seconds and repeat each stretch 2-3 times. It's important to stretch gently and avoid overstretching or bouncing, which can cause injury.

Building an Exercise Routine for Seniors Over 60

Building an exercise routine that is safe, effective, and enjoyable is key for seniors over 60. Here are some tips for building an exercise routine for seniors over 60:

Consult with a doctor: Seniors should consult with their doctor before starting any new exercise program, especially if they have any underlying health conditions or physical limitations.

Start slow: Seniors should start with short sessions of 10-15 minutes and gradually increase the duration and intensity of their workouts.

Choose exercises that are safe and appropriate.

Chapter 2

Types of exercises for seniors over 60

Regular exercise is important for everyone, regardless of age, and seniors over 60 can benefit greatly from incorporating exercise into their daily routine. Engaging in physical activity can help seniors maintain their mobility, independence, and overall health. However, it is important for seniors to choose exercises that are safe, low-impact, and appropriate for their fitness level. Here are some types of exercises that are suitable for seniors over 60:

Balance exercises: Falls are a major concern for seniors, so incorporating balance exercises into their routine is important for reducing the risk of falls. Exercises such as standing on one foot, heel-to-toe walks, and standing up from a chair without using hands can improve balance and stability.

It is important for seniors to consult with their doctor before starting an exercise routine and to start slowly, gradually increasing the intensity and duration of their workouts. Engaging in regular physical activity can help seniors stay healthy, independent, and active well into their golden years.

Low-impact cardio: Walking is a great form of low-impact cardio for seniors, but there are other options as well. Swimming is a particularly good choice for seniors as it is gentle on the joints and provides a full-body workout. Cycling, either on a stationary bike or outdoors, is another low-impact cardio option. Seniors should aim for at least 150 minutes of moderate-intensity aerobic activity per week, which can be broken up into smaller sessions throughout the day.

Strength training: Seniors should aim to do strength training exercises two to three times per week, focusing on all major muscle groups.

It is important to start with light weights or resistance bands and gradually increase the weight or resistance over time. Proper form is key to preventing injury, so it is important to work with a trainer or physical therapist to ensure proper technique.

Stretching and flexibility exercises: Seniors should aim to stretch daily to maintain flexibility and range of motion. Yoga and Pilates are great options for stretching and strengthening muscles. Seniors should start with gentle stretches and gradually increase the intensity over time. It is important to avoid bouncing during stretches, as this can cause injury.

Tai Chi: Tai Chi is a gentle, low-impact form of exercise that combines movement with mindfulness and deep breathing. It has been shown to improve balance, flexibility, and overall health in seniors. Tai Chi classes are often offered at community centers, senior centers, and fitness studios.

Chair exercises: Chair exercises are a great option for seniors who have mobility issues or difficulty standing for long periods of time. Seniors can do exercises such as seated leg lifts, arm curls, and seated marches while sitting in a chair.

In addition to the above exercises, seniors should also incorporate daily activities that keep them moving, such as gardening, housework, and taking walks. Seniors should also stay hydrated and listen to their body, taking breaks when needed and not pushing themselves too hard. Regular exercise can have numerous benefits for seniors, including improved physical and mental health, increased independence, and a higher quality of life.

Chapter 3

Building an exercise routine for seniors over 60

As we age, it becomes more important than ever to maintain a healthy and active lifestyle. Exercise is an essential component of healthy aging, providing numerous physical and mental health benefits. For seniors over the age of 60, creating an exercise routine that is safe, effective, and enjoyable can be challenging. However, with the right approach and a bit of guidance, seniors can develop a fitness plan that meets their unique needs and helps them achieve their health goals. In this article, we will provide tips and advice on how to build an exercise routine for seniors over 60 that is safe, effective, and enjoyable.

Consult with a healthcare professional

Before beginning any new exercise routine, seniors should consult with their healthcare professional. A doctor or physical therapist can assess a senior's current physical condition, identify any health concerns or limitations, and provide guidance on how to safely engage in physical activity. This is especially important for seniors who have pre-existing medical conditions or who are taking medications that may affect their ability to exercise safely.

Choose the right type of exercise
Seniors should choose exercises that are safe and appropriate for their fitness level and physical abilities. Low-impact activities such as walking, swimming, cycling, or yoga are generally safe and effective for seniors. Strength training exercises that focus on building muscle and bone density are also important for seniors. These exercises can be done with resistance bands or light weights, and they can help improve balance, reduce the risk of falls, and maintain independence.

Set realistic goals

Seniors should set realistic goals for their exercise routine. This can help keep them motivated and focused on their progress. Goals should be specific, measurable, and achievable. For example, a senior may set a goal to walk for 30 minutes a day, three days a week, or to lift a certain weight for a specific number of reps. Seniors should also track their progress and adjust their goals as needed.

Start slow and gradually increase intensity
Seniors should start with low-intensity exercises and gradually increase the intensity over time. This can help prevent injuries and minimize discomfort or soreness. Seniors should also warm up before exercising and cool down afterwards. A proper warm-up should include light stretching or gentle movements to increase blood flow and prepare the muscles for activity. A cool-down should include stretching exercises to help prevent stiffness and reduce the risk of injury.

Make it enjoyable
Seniors should choose activities that they enjoy and that fit their personality and lifestyle. This

can help them stay motivated and committed to their exercise routine. Seniors can join fitness classes or groups that cater to their interests, such as dance classes or outdoor walking groups. They can also listen to music or watch TV while exercising to make it more enjoyable.

Incorporate social support
Seniors can benefit from incorporating social support into their exercise routine. This can include exercising with friends or family members, joining a fitness class or group, or hiring a personal trainer. Social support can provide motivation, encouragement, and accountability, helping seniors stay committed to their exercise routine.

Stay hydrated and nourished
Seniors should stay hydrated before, during, and after exercise. Drinking water can help prevent dehydration and maintain energy levels. Seniors should also eat a balanced diet that provides the nutrients their body needs for physical activity. This can include protein to help build muscle, carbohydrates to provide

energy, and healthy fats to support overall health.

Listen to your body
Seniors should listen to their body and stop exercising if they experience pain or discomfort. They should also take breaks if they feel tired or fatigued. Over-exertion can increase the risk of injury and can be counterproductive to a senior's fitness goals.

Building an exercise routine for seniors over 60 requires a thoughtful approach.

Here is a sample exercise routine for seniors over 60 that includes a variety of exercises to improve strength, balance, flexibility, and cardiovascular fitness. It is important to note that this is just an example and seniors should adjust the exercises and intensity to their own abilities and fitness goals.

Exercise Type	Exercise	Sets/Reps	Intensity

Cardiovascular	Brisk walking	1 set of 10 minutes	Moderate
Balance	Single leg stance	3 sets of 30 seconds	Low to moderate
Strength	Bicep curl with resistance band	3 sets of 12 reps	Low to moderate
Flexibility	Seated hamstrin g stretch	3 sets of 30 seconds	Low
Cardiovascular	Stationar y bike	1 set of 10 minutes	Low to moderate
Balance	Side leg raise with chair support	3 sets of 12 reps(each side)	Low to moderate
Strength	Wall push-ups	3 sets of 12 reps	Low to moderate
Flexibility	Seated spinal twist	3 sets of 30 seconds (each	Low

		side)	
Cardiovascular	Swimming	1 set of 10 minutes	Low to moderate
Balance	Tandem stand with eyes closed	3 sets of 30 seconds	Low to moderate
Strength	Seated leg extension with ankle weights	3 sets of 12 reps	Low to moderate
Flexibility	Seated shoulder stretch	3 sets of 30 seconds (each side)	Low

Seniors can perform this routine two to three times per week, with at least one day of rest in between sessions. They can also add or modify exercises as they progress and adjust the intensity to their fitness level. It is important to start slow and gradually increase intensity over time. Additionally, seniors should always listen to their body and adjust the routine as needed.

Chapter 4

Incorporating technology into workouts for seniors over 60

As technology continues to evolve, it has become an increasingly important tool in helping seniors stay healthy and active. For seniors over 60, incorporating technology into their workout routines can provide numerous benefits, from tracking progress to increasing motivation and making exercise more accessible. In this article, we will discuss how technology can be used to enhance senior workouts, including the use of fitness apps, wearable devices, and online workout videos.

Fitness Apps
Fitness apps are becoming increasingly popular, and for good reason. They offer a wide

range of features, from tracking progress and setting goals to providing guidance and motivation. For seniors, fitness apps can be a valuable tool in helping them stay on track and achieve their fitness goals.

One popular fitness app is MyFitnessPal. This app allows seniors to track their food intake and exercise, making it easier for them to stay on top of their diet and exercise regimen. The app also provides personalized recommendations based on a user's goals and preferences, making it easier for seniors to stay motivated and on track.

Another popular fitness app is Fitbit. Fitbit is a wearable device that tracks steps taken, calories burned, and other metrics related to physical activity. The app also allows users to set goals and track progress, making it easier for seniors to stay motivated and on track.

Overall, fitness apps can be a valuable tool for seniors looking to incorporate technology into their workout routines. They provide personalized recommendations, tracking, and motivation, making it easier for seniors to achieve their fitness goals.

Wearable Devices

Wearable devices are another popular option for seniors looking to incorporate technology into their workout routines. These devices can track a wide range of metrics, from heart rate and steps taken to calories burned and sleep quality. They can also provide personalized recommendations and reminders, making it easier for seniors to stay on track.

One popular wearable device for seniors is the Apple Watch. The Apple Watch tracks physical activity, heart rate, and other metrics related to fitness. It also offers personalized coaching and motivation, making it easier for seniors to stay on track and achieve their fitness goals.

Another popular wearable device is the Fitbit. The Fitbit tracks steps taken, calories burned, and other metrics related to physical activity. It also offers personalized coaching and motivation, making it easier for seniors to stay on track and achieve their fitness goals.

Overall, wearable devices can be a valuable tool for seniors looking to incorporate technology into their workout routines. They provide personalized recommendations, tracking, and motivation, making it easier for seniors to achieve their fitness goals.

Online Workout Videos
Online workout videos are another popular option for seniors looking to incorporate technology into their workout routines. These videos offer a wide range of workouts, from yoga and Pilates to cardio and strength training. They can be accessed from anywhere, making it easier for seniors to workout on their own time and at their own pace.

One popular online workout video platform is YouTube. YouTube offers a wide range of workout videos, from beginner to advanced. These videos can be accessed for free, making it an affordable option for seniors on a budget.

Another popular online workout video platform is Peloton. Peloton offers live and on-demand workout classes, including cycling, yoga, and strength training. While Peloton does require a monthly subscription fee, it offers personalized coaching and motivation, making it a valuable tool for seniors looking to stay motivated and achieve their fitness goals.

Overall, online workout videos can be a valuable tool for seniors looking to incorporate technology into their workout routines. They offer a wide range of workouts, personalized coaching, and can be accessed from anywhere, making it easier for seniors to stay on track and achieve their fitness goals.

Benefits of Incorporating Technology into Workouts for Seniors Over 60
Incorporating technology into workouts for seniors over 60 can provide numerous benefits. Some of these benefits include:

There are many benefits to incorporating technology into workouts for seniors over 60. Some of the key advantages are:

Improved motivation: Technology can provide a fun and engaging way to exercise, which can motivate seniors to stick to their fitness routines.

Increased accessibility: Technology can make exercise more accessible for seniors who may have mobility issues or live in areas where outdoor exercise isn't feasible. For example, there are many online workout programs and apps that seniors can use to exercise in the comfort of their own homes.

Better tracking: Technology can help seniors track their progress and monitor their health. For example, fitness trackers can measure heart rate, steps taken, and calories burned, which can provide valuable data for seniors to monitor their fitness levels.

Personalization: Technology can help seniors customize their workouts to meet their individual needs and fitness goals. For example, many workout apps offer personalized workout plans based on the user's fitness level and goals.

Social connection: Technology can help seniors connect with others who share their fitness goals and interests. For example, there are many online fitness communities and social media groups where seniors can share tips, advice, and encouragement with others.

Incorporating technology into workouts can provide seniors with a convenient, engaging, and effective way to stay fit and healthy.

Chapter 5

Working out with chronic health conditions

Regular physical activity is essential for individuals of all ages, including seniors with chronic health conditions. However, it is important to note that not all types of exercise or workouts are suitable for seniors with chronic health conditions. Seniors with chronic health conditions may need to modify their workouts to suit their needs and improve their health. In this article, we will discuss how seniors with chronic health conditions can modify their workouts to suit their needs and improve their health.

Chronic health conditions that affect seniors can include arthritis, osteoporosis, heart disease, and diabetes, among others. Exercise and physical activity can help seniors with these conditions to manage their symptoms, maintain their independence, and improve their overall health and well-being. However, seniors with chronic health conditions should be cautious when starting or modifying their workout routines.

Here are some tips on how seniors with chronic health conditions can modify their workouts to suit their needs and improve their health:

Consult with a healthcare professional
Before starting any new workout routine or modifying an existing one, seniors with chronic health conditions should consult with a healthcare professional. A healthcare professional can help seniors to determine which types of exercise and physical activity are safe for them based on their health condition, current fitness level, and medical history. A healthcare professional can also help seniors to set realistic goals and develop a workout plan that suits their needs and abilities.

Choose low-impact exercises
Seniors with chronic health conditions may need to choose low-impact exercises that are easier on their joints and muscles. Low-impact exercises can include walking, cycling, swimming, water aerobics, yoga, tai chi, and Pilates. These exercises can help seniors to improve their cardiovascular health, flexibility, strength, and balance without putting too much stress on their bodies.

Incorporate strength training
Strength training is essential for seniors with chronic health conditions, as it can help to improve muscle strength, bone density, and joint flexibility. Seniors with chronic health conditions should start with light weights or resistance bands and gradually increase the intensity as they become stronger. Strength training exercises can include bicep curls, squats, lunges, and shoulder presses.

Warm up and cool down
Seniors with chronic health conditions should always warm up and cool down before and after exercise to prevent injury and reduce muscle

soreness. A warm-up can include light cardio exercises, such as walking or cycling, and gentle stretches. A cool-down can include slower-paced exercises, such as walking or stretching, to gradually lower the heart rate and reduce muscle tension.

Monitor intensity
Seniors with chronic health conditions should monitor their exercise intensity to prevent overexertion and injury. Exercise intensity can be measured using a heart rate monitor or by monitoring the rate of perceived exertion (RPE). The RPE scale ranges from 1 to 10, with 1 being very light and 10 being very hard. Seniors with chronic health conditions should aim for an RPE of 4-6, which is moderate intensity.

Stay hydrated
Seniors with chronic health conditions should stay hydrated during exercise to prevent dehydration and overheating. Drinking water before, during, and after exercise can help to maintain proper hydration levels. Seniors with chronic health conditions should also avoid

exercising in extreme temperatures, such as hot or cold weather, as it can be harmful to their health.

Listen to your body
Seniors with chronic health conditions should listen to their bodies and adjust their workout routines accordingly. If they experience pain, discomfort, or shortness of breath, they should stop exercising and seek medical attention if necessary. Seniors with chronic health conditions should also avoid pushing themselves too hard and take breaks as needed.

Seniors with chronic health conditions can modify their workouts to suit their needs and improve their health.

By consulting with a healthcare professional, choosing low-impact exercises, incorporating strength training, warming up and cooling down, monitoring intensity, staying hydrated, and listening to their bodies, seniors with chronic health conditions can safely and effectively improve their overall health and well-being through regular physical activity.

It is important to note that seniors with chronic health conditions may have limitations that require additional modifications to their workouts. For example, seniors with arthritis may need to avoid high-impact exercises that can put stress on their joints, while seniors with heart disease may need to avoid exercises that increase their heart rate too much. Seniors with chronic health conditions should work closely with their healthcare provider to determine the best exercises and modifications for their individual needs.

In addition to modifying their workouts, seniors with chronic health conditions should also prioritize proper nutrition, adequate rest, and stress management to support their overall health and well-being. By taking a holistic approach to their health, seniors with chronic health conditions can improve their quality of life and maintain their independence as they age.

Regular physical activity is essential for seniors with chronic health conditions to manage their symptoms, maintain their independence, and improve their overall health and well-being. By modifying their workouts to suit their needs and abilities, seniors with chronic health conditions can safely and effectively improve their physical fitness and health. Consultation with a healthcare professional, choosing low-impact exercises, incorporating strength training, warming up and cooling down, monitoring intensity, staying hydrated, and listening to their bodies are all important steps for seniors with chronic health conditions to take when starting or modifying their workout routines.

Chapter 6

Staying motivated to exercise as a senior

As we age, it becomes increasingly important to maintain an active and healthy lifestyle. Exercise has been shown to improve physical health, reduce the risk of chronic diseases, and enhance mental well-being. However, many seniors struggle to stay motivated and committed to their exercise routine, which can lead to a sedentary lifestyle and a decline in health. In this article, we will explore some tips and strategies for seniors to stay motivated and committed to their exercise routine.

Find an Exercise Buddy:
One of the most effective ways to stay motivated and committed to an exercise routine is to find an exercise buddy. Having a partner to exercise

with can make the experience more enjoyable, provide accountability, and help seniors stay motivated. It can also provide an opportunity for socialization, which is important for mental well-being.

There are several ways to find an exercise buddy. Seniors can ask a friend or family member to exercise with them, join a group fitness class, or join a local walking or running club. There are also online resources, such as Meetup and SilverSneakers, which can help seniors connect with others who share their interests.

Set Achievable Goals:
Setting achievable goals is an important part of staying motivated and committed to an exercise routine. Seniors should set goals that are realistic and attainable, based on their current fitness level and health status. For example, a senior who has not exercised in several years may start with a goal of walking for 10 minutes per day and gradually increase the duration and intensity of their exercise over time.

It is also important to track progress toward goals. Seniors can use a fitness tracker or journal to record their workouts, measure their progress, and celebrate their successes. Tracking progress can provide a sense of accomplishment and motivation to continue with an exercise routine.

Try New Activities:
Trying new activities can help seniors stay motivated and engaged with their exercise routine. Seniors may find that they enjoy certain activities more than others, which can help them stay committed to their exercise routine.

There are many different types of exercise that seniors can try, such as yoga, Pilates, swimming, cycling, and strength training. Seniors can also try different types of group fitness classes, such as Zumba, dance classes, or water aerobics. Trying new activities can also provide opportunities for socialization and meeting new people.

Make Exercise a Part of Daily Routine:

Making exercise a part of daily routine can help seniors stay committed to their exercise routine. Seniors should aim to incorporate physical activity into their daily routine, such as taking a daily walk after dinner, doing a few stretches in the morning, or taking the stairs instead of the elevator.

It is important to find activities that are enjoyable and can be sustained over the long-term. Seniors should aim to find an exercise routine that fits their lifestyle and preferences, and that can be easily incorporated into their daily routine.

Find a Professional Trainer:
Finding a professional trainer can help seniors stay motivated and committed to their exercise routine. A professional trainer can provide guidance and support, create a personalized exercise plan, and provide accountability.

There are several different types of professional trainers, such as personal trainers, physical therapists, and fitness instructors. Seniors should choose a trainer who is experienced in

working with seniors and who understands
their unique needs and limitations.

Focus on the Benefits:
Focusing on the benefits of exercise can help
seniors stay motivated and committed to their
exercise routine. Exercise has many physical
and mental health benefits, such as improved
cardiovascular health, increased strength and
flexibility, reduced risk of chronic diseases, and
enhanced mood and well-being.

Seniors should focus on the positive changes
that exercise can bring to their life, and use
these benefits as motivation to continue with
their exercise routine.

Overcome Barriers:
There are often barriers that seniors face when
trying to maintain an exercise routine. Some
common barriers include lack of motivation,
physical limitations, and chronic health
conditions. Seniors can overcome these barriers
by finding ways to adapt their exercise routine
to their unique needs and limitations.

For example, seniors with physical limitations can work with a physical therapist to develop an exercise plan that accommodates their needs. Seniors with chronic health conditions can work with their healthcare provider to develop a safe and effective exercise plan that addresses their specific health needs.

You can also find ways to make exercise more enjoyable and engaging. This may involve listening to music while exercising, watching TV or movies during workouts, or finding a workout buddy or group.

Celebrate Successes
Celebrating successes can help seniors stay motivated and committed to their exercise routine. Seniors should celebrate their successes, no matter how small they may be. This can provide a sense of accomplishment and motivation to continue with an exercise routine.

Seniors can celebrate their successes by treating themselves to a special meal or activity, sharing

their progress with friends and family, or
rewarding themselves with a small gift.

Staying motivated and committed to an exercise
routine is important for seniors to maintain
physical and mental health. Seniors can find
motivation and support by finding an exercise
buddy, setting achievable goals, trying new
activities, making exercise a part of their daily
routine, finding a professional trainer, focusing
on the benefits of exercise, overcoming barriers,
and celebrating successes. By incorporating
these tips and strategies, you can maintain an
active and healthy lifestyle for years to come

Chapter 7

Overcoming barriers to exercise for seniors over 60

As people age, physical activity becomes increasingly important for maintaining health and well-being. Regular exercise can help seniors maintain mobility, prevent chronic diseases, and improve mental health. However, many seniors face barriers that prevent them from exercising regularly. Common barriers include fear of injury, lack of motivation, and physical limitations. In this essay, we will address these barriers and offer advice on how seniors can overcome them.

Fear of Injury:

Fear of injury is a common barrier to exercise for seniors. As people age, the risk of falls and injuries increases, and many seniors worry that exercising will put them at greater risk. However, avoiding exercise altogether can actually increase the risk of injury by causing muscle weakness and stiffness.

To overcome the fear of injury, seniors should start with low-impact exercises that are less likely to cause injury. Walking, swimming, and yoga are all great options. Seniors should also consult with their doctor before starting a new exercise routine to make sure they are healthy enough for physical activity. Starting slowly and gradually increasing the intensity and duration of exercise can also help build confidence and reduce the risk of injury.

Lack of Motivation:

Lack of motivation is another common barrier to exercise for seniors. Many seniors find it difficult to stay motivated to exercise, especially if they do not enjoy the activity or do not see immediate results.

To overcome lack of motivation, seniors should find an exercise they enjoy. This could be anything from dancing to gardening to taking a daily walk. Seniors should also set goals for themselves and track their progress. This can help them see the results of their hard work and stay motivated. Exercising with friends or family members can also be a great way to stay motivated and make exercise more enjoyable.

Physical Limitations:

Physical limitations can also be a barrier to exercise for seniors. Arthritis, joint pain, and other physical conditions can make certain types of exercise difficult or even impossible.

To overcome physical limitations, seniors should focus on exercises that are safe and appropriate for their physical condition. This may mean avoiding high-impact exercises that put stress on joints and focusing on low-impact exercises like swimming or cycling. Seniors should also consider working with a physical therapist or personal trainer who can help them develop a safe and effective exercise routine that takes into account their physical limitations.

Other Tips for Overcoming Barriers to Exercise:

In addition to addressing the specific barriers outlined above, there are several other tips that can help seniors overcome barriers to exercise:

Make exercise a priority: Seniors should prioritize exercise and make it a regular part of their routine. This may mean scheduling exercise at the same time every day or finding a gym or fitness class that fits their schedule.

Stay hydrated: Drinking plenty of water before, during, and after exercise can help seniors stay hydrated and prevent fatigue.

Wear appropriate clothing and footwear: Seniors should wear comfortable, supportive clothing and footwear that is appropriate for the type of exercise they are doing.

Take breaks when needed: It is important for seniors to listen to their bodies and take breaks when needed. If they feel tired or in pain, they should rest and take a break from exercise.

Get enough rest: Seniors should make sure they are getting enough rest and sleep to support their exercise routine.

Stay positive: Finally, it is important for seniors to stay positive and focus on the benefits of exercise. Regular exercise can improve mood, reduce stress, and increase overall well-being.

In conclusion, there are several common barriers that prevent seniors from exercising regularly, including fear of injury, lack of motivation, and physical limitations. However, with the right strategies and support, seniors can overcome these barriers and enjoy the many benefits of regular exercise. By starting slowly, finding an exercise they enjoy, and working with a physical therapist or personal trainer, seniors can develop

www.ingramcontent.com/pod-product-compliance
Lightning Source LLC
Chambersburg PA
CBHW061606250726
48657CB00017B/2156